Mediterranean
Diet

The Ultimate Guide to the Mediterranean Diet with Recipes

Helen Howard

TABLE OF CONTANTS

INTRODUCTION

The Mediterranean Diet is a diet that is rich in plant-based foods, like vegetables, fruits, nuts, seeds, beans and legumes, and olive oil. These foods are high in antioxidants, which are compounds that can protect your cells from damage. The Mediterranean diet is also high in fibre, which is a nutrient that helps keep your digestive system healthy. The Mediterranean diet has been shown to reduce the risk of heart disease, cancer, stroke, and Alzheimer's. It's also been shown to reduce the risk of cognitive decline, increase longevity, and improve mood and memory

That's how the Mediterranean "diet" becomes a Mediterranean "lifestyle" that closely resembles the people of the region. Greece's citizens lead an active lifestyle, engaging in some kind of physical activity on a regular basis. Reading, sailing, rowing, swimming, or hiking are all examples of physical activity that can be combined with a balanced plant-based diet to produce positive health outcomes. Physical exercise in today's world could include a trip to the gym or even a simple walk around the street. It doesn't have to be strenuous; the main thing is to include some kind of physical activity in your day so that you can reap the full benefits of this diet.

Before we get into a basic list of what you can and can't eat, it's important to note that the Mediterranean region is made up of several nations, each with its own distinct dietary preferences.

With this variety comes a wide range of recipes that you can use in your dishes as long as you stick to the Mediterranean diet's balanced principles. This gives you a general idea of which foods to include on your shopping list, and then you can start looking for recipes! What does a typical Mediterranean diet entail?

Whole grain bread, extra virgin olive oil, fresh fruits and vegetables, herbs and spices, nuts and seeds, fish and seafood can all be part of your diet. Poultry, cheese, eggs, and yogurt should be consumed in moderation.

· Red meat and organ meat should be consumed in moderation. Processed snacks, refined oils (canola or palm oil), refined grains (white bread), sugary beverages (juice, soda), processed meats (hot dogs, sausages, bacon), and trans fats should all be avoided.

· Water and wine should be consumed.

BREAKFAST RECIPES

1. Savory Muffins

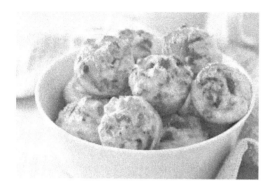

Preparation time: 9 minutes

Cooking Time: 15 minutes

Serving: 6

Ingredients

- 9 ham slices
- 1/3 c. chopped spinach
- ¼ c. crumbled feta cheese
- ½ c. chopped roasted red peppers
- Salt and black pepper
- 1½ tbsps. basil pesto
- 5 whisked eggs

Direction

1. Grease a muffin tin. Use 1 ½ ham slices to line each of the muffin molds.
2. Except for black pepper, salt, pesto, and eggs, divide the rest of the ingredients into your ham cups.
3. Using a bowl, whisk together the pepper, salt, pesto, and eggs. Pour your pepper mixture on top.
4. Set oven to 400 F/204 C and bake for about 15 minutes.
5. Serve immediately.

Nutrition 109 Calories 6.7g Fat 9.3g Protein

2. Farro Salad

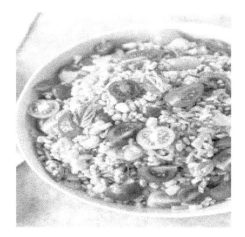

Preparation Time: 7 minutes

Cooking Time: 5 minutes

Serving: 2

Ingredient

- 1 tbsp. olive oil

- Salt and black pepper

- 1 bunch baby spinach, chopped

- 1 pitted avocado, peeled and chopped

- 1 minced garlic clove

- 2 c. cooked farro

- ½ c. cherry tomatoes, cubed

Direction

1. Adjust your heat to medium. Set oil in a pan and heat.
2. Toss in the rest of the ingredients. Cook the mixture for approximately 5 minutes.
3. Set in serving plates and enjoy.

Nutrition 157 Calories 13.7g Fat 3.6g Protein

3. Cranberry and Dates Squares

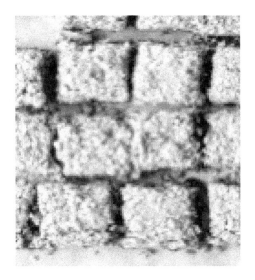

Preparation Time: 9 minutes

Cooking Time: 30 minutes

Serving: 10

Ingredients

- 12 pitted dates, chopped

- 1 tsp. vanilla extract

- ¼ c. honey

- ½ c. rolled oats

- ¾ c. dried cranberries

- ¼ c. melted almond avocado oil

- 1 c. chopped walnuts, roasted

- ¼ c. pumpkin seeds

Direction

1. Using a bowl, stir in all ingredients to mix.
2. Line a parchment paper on a baking sheet. Press the mixture on the setup.
3. Set in your freezer for about 30 minutes. Slice into 10 squares and enjoy.

Nutrition 263 Calories 13.4g Fat 3.5g Protein

4. Lentils and Cheddar Frittata

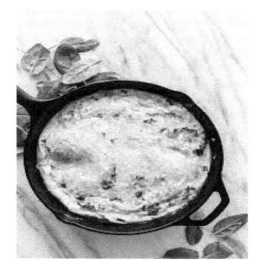

Preparation Time: 4 minutes

Cooking Time: 17 minutes

Serving: 4

Ingredients

- 1 chopped red onion

- 2 tbsps. olive oil

- 1 c. boiled sweet potatoes, chopped

- ¾ c. chopped ham

- 4 whisked eggs

- ¾ c. cooked lentils

- 2 tbsps. Greek yogurt

- Salt and black pepper

- ½ c. halved cherry tomatoes,

- ¾ c. grated cheddar cheese

Direction

1. Adjust your heat to medium and set a pan in place. Add in oil to heat. Stir in onion and allow to sauté for about 2 minutes.
2. Except for cheese and eggs, toss in the other ingredients and cook for 3 more minutes.
4. Add in the eggs, top with cheese. Cook for 10 more minutes while covered.
5. Slice the frittata, set in serving bowls and enjoy.

Nutrition 274 Calories 17.36g Fat 11.4g Protein

5. Tuna Sandwich

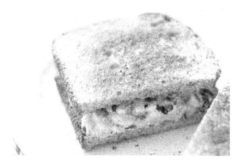

Preparation Time: 9 minutes

Cooking Time: 5 minutes

Serving: 2

Ingredients

- 6 oz. canned tuna, drained and flaked

- 1 pitted avocado, peeled and mashed

- 4 whole-wheat bread slices

- Pinch salt and black pepper

- 1 tbsp. crumbled feta cheese

- 1 c. baby spinach

Direction

1. Using a bowl, stir in pepper, salt, tuna, and cheese to mix.

2. To the bread slices, apply a spread of the mashed avocado.

3.   Equally, divide the tuna mixture and spinach onto 2 of the slices. Top with the remaining 2 slices. Serve.

Nutrition 283 Calories 11.2g Fat 4.5g Protein

6. Mediterranean Pita Breakfast

Preparation Time: 22 minutes

Cooking Time: 3 minutes

Servings: 2

Ingredients:

- 1/4 cup of sweet red pepper
- 1/4 cup of chopped onion
- 1 cup of egg substitute
- 1/8 teaspoon of salt
- 1/8 teaspoon of pepper
- 1 small chopped tomato
- 1/2 cup of fresh torn baby spinach
- 1-1/2 teaspoons of minced fresh basil
- 2 whole size pita breads
- 2 tablespoons of crumbled feta cheese

Directions:

1. Coat with a cooking spray a small size non-stick skillet. Stir in the onion and red pepper for 3 minutes over medium heat.
2. Add your egg substitute and season with salt and pepper. Stir cook until it sets. Mix the torn spinach, chopped tomatoes, and mince basil. Scoop onto the pitas. Top vegetable mixture with your egg mixture.

3. Topped with crumbled feta cheese and serve immediately.

Nutrition 267 Calories 3g Fat 20g Protein

7. Hummus Deviled Egg

Preparation Time: 10 minutes

Cooking Time: 0 minute

Servings: 6

Ingredients:

- 1/4 cup of finely diced cucumber
- 1/4 cup of finely diced tomato
- 2 teaspoons of fresh lemon juice
- 1/8 teaspoon salt
- 6 hard-cooked peeled eggs, sliced half lengthwise
- 1/3 cup of roasted garlic hummus or any hummus flavor
- Chopped fresh parsley (optional)

Directions:

1. Combine the tomato, lemon juice, cucumber and salt together and then gently mix. Scrape out the yolks from the halved eggs and store for later use. Scoop a heaping teaspoon of humus in each half egg. Top with parsley and half-teaspoon tomato-cucumber mixture. Serve immediately

Nutrition 40 Calories 1g Fat 4g Protein

8. Smoked Salmon Scrambled Egg

Preparation Time: 2 minutes

Cooking Time: 8 minutes

Servings: 4

Ingredients:

- 16 ounces egg substitute, cholesterol-free
- 1/8 teaspoon of black pepper
- 2 tablespoons of sliced green onions, keep the tops
- 1 ounce of chilled reduced-fat cream cheese, cut into 1/4-inch cubes
- 2 ounces of flaked smoked salmon

Directions:

1. Cut the chilled cream cheese into ¼-inch cubes then set aside. Whisk the egg substitute and the pepper in a large sized bowl Coat a non-stick skillet with cooking spray over medium heat. Stir in the egg substitute and cook for 5 to 7 minutes or until it starts to set stirring occasionally and scraping bottom of the pan.
2. Fold in the cream cheese, green onions and the salmon. Continue cooking then stir for another 3 minutes or just until the eggs are still moist but cooked.

Nutrition 100 Calories 3g Fats 15g Protein

9. Buckwheat Apple-Raisin Muffin

Preparation Time: 24 minutes

Cooking Time: 20 minutes

Servings: 12

Ingredients:

- 1 cup of all-purpose flour
- 3/4 cup of buckwheat flour
- 2 tablespoons of brown sugar
- 1 1/2 teaspoons of baking powder
- 1/4 teaspoon of baking soda
- 3/4 cup of reduced-fat buttermilk
- 2 tablespoons of olive oil
- 1 large egg
- 1 cup peeled and cored, fresh diced apples
- 1/4 cup of golden raisins

Directions:

1. Prepare the oven at 375 degrees F. Line a 12-cup muffin tin with a non-stick cooking spray or paper cups. Set aside. Incorporate all the dry ingredients in a mixing bowl. Set aside.

2. Beat together the liquid ingredients until smooth. Transfer the liquid mixture over the flour mixture and mix until moistened. Fold in the diced apples and raisins. Fill each muffin cups with about 2/3 full of the

mixture. Bake until it turns golden brown. Use the toothpick test. Serve.

Nutrition 117 Calories 1g Fat 3g Protein

10. Pumpkin Bran Muffin

Preparation Time: 20 minutes

Cooking Time: 20 minutes

Servings: 22

Ingredients:

- 3/4 cup of all-purpose flour
- 3/4 cup of whole wheat flour
- 2 tablespoons sugar
- 1 tablespoon of baking powder
- 1/8 teaspoon salt
- 1 teaspoon of pumpkin pie spice
- 2 cups of 100% bran cereal
- 1 1/2 cups of skim milk
- 2 egg whites
- 15 ounces x 1 can pumpkin
- 2 tablespoons of avocado oil

Directions:

1. Preheat the oven to 400 degrees Fahrenheit. Prepare a muffin pan enough for 22 muffins and line with a non-stick cooking spray. Stir together the first four ingredients until combined. Set aside.
2. Using a large mixing bowl, mix together milk and cereal bran and let it stand for 2 minutes or until the cereal softens. Add in the oil, egg whites, and pumpkin in the bran mix and blend well. Fill in the flour mixture and mix well.

3. Divide the batter into equal portions into the muffin pan. Bake for 20 minutes. Pull out the muffins from pan and serve warm or cooled.

Nutrition 70 Calories 3g Fat 3g Protein

APPETIZERS AND SNACKS

11. Savory Muffins

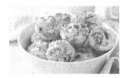

Preparation time: 9 minutes

Cooking Time: 15 minutes

Serving: 6

Ingredients

- 9 ham slices

- 1/3 c. chopped spinach

- ¼ c. crumbled feta cheese

- ½ c. chopped roasted red peppers

- Salt and black pepper

- 1½ tbsps. basil pesto

- 5 whisked eggs

Direction

1. Grease a muffin tin. Use 1 ½ ham slices to line each of the muffin molds.
2. Except for black pepper, salt, pesto, and eggs, divide the rest of the ingredients into your ham cups.

3. Using a bowl, whisk together the pepper, salt, pesto, and eggs. Pour your pepper mixture on top.
4. Set oven to 400 F/204 C and bake for about 15 minutes.
5. Serve immediately.

Nutrition 109 Calories 6.7g Fat 9.3g Protein

12. Farro Salad

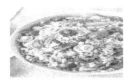

Preparation Time: 7 minutes

Cooking Time: 5 minutes

Serving: 2

Ingredient

- 1 tbsp. olive oil
- Salt and black pepper
- 1 bunch baby spinach, chopped
- 1 pitted avocado, peeled and chopped
- 1 minced garlic clove
- 2 c. cooked farro
- ½ c. cherry tomatoes, cubed

Direction

1. Adjust your heat to medium. Set oil in a pan and heat.
3. Toss in the rest of the ingredients. Cook the mixture for approximately 5 minutes.
4. Set in serving plates and enjoy.

Nutrition 157 Calories 13.7g Fat 3.6g Protein

13. Cranberry and Dates Squares

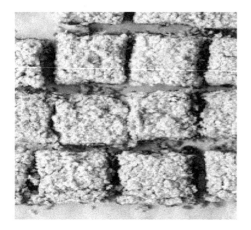

Preparation Time: 9 minutes

Cooking Time: 30 minutes

Serving: 10

Ingredients

- 12 pitted dates, chopped
- 1 tsp. vanilla extract
- ¼ c. honey
- ½ c. rolled oats
- ¾ c. dried cranberries
- ¼ c. melted almond avocado oil
- 1 c. chopped walnuts, roasted
- ¼ c. pumpkin seeds

Direction

1. Using a bowl, stir in all ingredients to mix.
2. Line a parchment paper on a baking sheet. Press the mixture on the setup.
3. Set in your freezer for about 30 minutes. Slice into 10 squares and enjoy.

Nutrition 263 Calories 13.4g Fat 3.5g Protein

14. Lentils and Cheddar Frittata

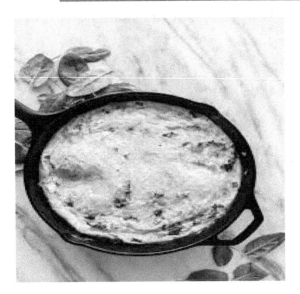

Preparation Time: 4 minutes

Cooking Time: 17 minutes

Serving: 4

Ingredients

- 1 chopped red onion

- 2 tbsps. olive oil

- 1 c. boiled sweet potatoes, chopped

- ¾ c. chopped ham

- 4 whisked eggs

- ¾ c. cooked lentils

- 2 tbsps. Greek yogurt

- Salt and black pepper

- ½ c. halved cherry tomatoes,
- ¾ c. grated cheddar cheese

Direction

1. Adjust your heat to medium and set a pan in place. Add in oil to heat. Stir in onion and allow to sauté for about 2 minutes.
2. Except for cheese and eggs, toss in the other ingredients and cook for 3 more minutes.
3. Add in the eggs, top with cheese. Cook for 10 more minutes while covered.
4. Slice the frittata, set in serving bowls and enjoy.

Nutrition 274 Calories 17.36g Fat 11.4g Protein

15. Tuna Sandwich

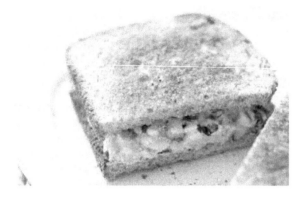

Preparation Time: 9 minutes

Cooking Time: 5 minutes

Serving: 2

Ingredients

- 6 oz. canned tuna, drained and flaked
- 1 pitted avocado, peeled and mashed
- 4 whole-wheat bread slices
- Pinch salt and black pepper
- 1 tbsp. crumbled feta cheese
- 1 c. baby spinach

Direction

1. Using a bowl, stir in pepper, salt, tuna, and cheese to mix.
2. To the bread slices, apply a spread of the mashed avocado.

3. Equally, divide the tuna mixture and spinach onto 2 of the slices. Top with the remaining 2 slices. Serve.

Nutrition 283 Calories 11.2g Fat 4.5g Protein

16. Mediterranean Pita Breakfast

Preparation Time: 22 minutes

Cooking Time: 3 minutes

Servings: 2

Ingredients:

- 1/4 cup of sweet red pepper
- 1/4 cup of chopped onion
- 1 cup of egg substitute
- 1/8 teaspoon of salt
- 1/8 teaspoon of pepper
- 1 small chopped tomato
- 1/2 cup of fresh torn baby spinach
- 1-1/2 teaspoons of minced fresh basil
- 2 whole size pita breads
- 2 tablespoons of crumbled feta cheese

Directions:

1. Coat with a cooking spray a small size non-stick skillet. Stir in the onion and red pepper for 3 minutes over medium heat.
2. Add your egg substitute and season with salt and pepper. Stir cook until it sets. Mix the torn spinach, chopped tomatoes, and mince basil. Scoop onto the pitas. Top vegetable mixture with your egg mixture.

3. Topped with crumbled feta cheese and serve immediately.

Nutrition 267 Calories 3g Fat 20g Protein

17. Hummus Deviled Egg

Preparation Time: 10 minutes

Cooking Time: 0 minute

Servings: 6

Ingredients:

- 1/4 cup of finely diced cucumber
- 1/4 cup of finely diced tomato
- 2 teaspoons of fresh lemon juice
- 1/8 teaspoon salt
- 6 hard-cooked peeled eggs, sliced half lengthwise
- 1/3 cup of roasted garlic hummus or any hummus flavor
- Chopped fresh parsley (optional)

Directions:

1. Combine the tomato, lemon juice, cucumber and salt together and then gently mix. Scrape out the yolks from the halved eggs and store for later use. Scoop a heaping teaspoon of humus in each half egg. Top with parsley and half-teaspoon tomato-cucumber mixture. Serve immediately

Nutrition 40 Calories 1g Fat 4g Protein

18. Smoked Salmon Scrambled Egg

Preparation Time: 2 minutes

Cooking Time: 8 minutes

Servings: 4

Ingredients:

- 16 ounces egg substitute, cholesterol-free
- 1/8 teaspoon of black pepper
- 2 tablespoons of sliced green onions, keep the tops
- 1 ounce of chilled reduced-fat cream cheese, cut into 1/4-inch cubes
- 2 ounces of flaked smoked salmon

Directions:

1. Cut the chilled cream cheese into ¼-inch cubes then set aside. Whisk the egg substitute and the pepper in a large sized bowl Coat a non-stick skillet with cooking spray over medium heat. Stir in the egg substitute and cook for 5 to 7 minutes or until it starts to set stirring occasionally and scraping bottom of the pan.
2. Fold in the cream cheese, green onions and the salmon. Continue cooking then stir for another 3 minutes or just until the eggs are still moist but cooked.

Nutrition 100 Calories 3g Fats 15g Protein

19. Buckwheat Apple-Raisin Muffin

Preparation Time: 24 minutes

Cooking Time: 20 minutes

Servings: 12

Ingredients:

- 1 cup of all-purpose flour
- 3/4 cup of buckwheat flour
- 2 tablespoons of brown sugar
- 1 1/2 teaspoons of baking powder
- 1/4 teaspoon of baking soda
- 3/4 cup of reduced-fat buttermilk
- 2 tablespoons of olive oil
- 1 large egg
- 1 cup peeled and cored, fresh diced apples
- 1/4 cup of golden raisins

Directions:

1. Prepare the oven at 375 degrees F. Line a 12-cup muffin tin with a non-stick cooking spray or paper cups. Set aside. Incorporate all the dry ingredients in a mixing bowl. Set aside.

2. Beat together the liquid ingredients until smooth. Transfer the liquid mixture over the flour mixture and mix until moistened. Fold in the diced apples and

raisins. Fill each muffin cups with about 2/3 full of the mixture. Bake until it turns golden brown. Use the toothpick test. Serve.

Nutrition 117 Calories 1g Fat 3g Protein

20. Pumpkin Bran Muffin

Preparation Time: 20 minutes

Cooking Time: 20 minutes

Servings: 22

Ingredients:

- 3/4 cup of all-purpose flour
- 3/4 cup of whole wheat flour
- 2 tablespoons sugar
- 1 tablespoon of baking powder
- 1/8 teaspoon salt
- 1 teaspoon of pumpkin pie spice
- 2 cups of 100% bran cereal
- 1 1/2 cups of skim milk
- 2 egg whites
- 15 ounces x 1 can pumpkin
- 2 tablespoons of avocado oil

Directions:

1. Preheat the oven to 400 degrees Fahrenheit. Prepare a muffin pan enough for 22 muffins and line with a non-stick cooking spray. Stir together the first four ingredients until combined. Set aside.
2. Using a large mixing bowl, mix together milk and cereal bran and let it stand for 2 minutes or until the cereal softens. Add in the oil, egg whites, and pumpkin in the bran mix and blend well. Fill in the flour mixture and mix well.

3. Divide the batter into equal portions into the muffin pan. Bake for 20 minutes. Pull out the muffins from pan and serve warm or cooled.

Nutrition 70 Calories 3g Fat 3g Protein

21. Perfect Pizza

Preparation Time: 35 minutes

Cooking Time: 15 minutes

Servings: 10

Ingredients:

For the Pizza Dough:

- 2-tsp honey
- 1/4-oz. active dry yeast
- 11/4-cups warm water (about 120 °F)
- 2-tbsp olive oil
- 1-tsp sea salt
- 3-cups whole grain flour + 1/4-cup, as needed for rolling

For the Pizza Topping:

- 1-cup pesto sauce
- 1-cup artichoke hearts
- 1-cup wilted spinach leaves
- 1-cup sun-dried tomato
- 1/2-cup Kalamata olives
- 4-oz. feta cheese
- 4-oz. mixed cheese of equal parts low-fat mozzarella, asiago, and provolone Olive oil

Optional Topping Add-Ons:

- Bell pepper
- Chicken breast, strips Fresh basil
- Pine nuts

Directions:

For the Pizza Dough:

1. Preheat your oven to 350 °F.
2. Stir the honey and yeast with the warm water in your food processor with a dough attachment. Blend the mixture until fully combined. Let the mixture to rest for 5 minutes to ensure the activity of the yeast through the appearance of bubbles on the surface.
3. Pour in the olive oil. Add the salt, and blend for half a minute. Add gradually 3 cups of flour, about half a cup at a time, blending for a couple of minutes between each addition.
4. Let your processor knead the mixture for 10 minutes until smooth and elastic, sprinkling it with flour whenever necessary to prevent the dough from sticking to the processor bowl's surfaces.
5. Take the dough from the bowl. Let it stand for 15 minutes, covered with a moist, warm towel.
6. Roll out the dough to a half-inch thickness, dusting it with flour as needed. Poke holes indiscriminately on the dough using a fork to prevent crust bubbling.
7. Place the perforated, rolled dough on a pizza stone or baking sheet. Bake for 5 minutes.

For the Pizza Topping:

8. Lightly brush the baked pizza shell with olive oil.
9. Pour over the pesto sauce and spread thoroughly over the pizza shell's surface, leaving out a half-inch space around its edge as the crust.
10. Top the pizza with artichoke hearts, wilted spinach leaves, sun-dried tomatoes, and olives. (Top with more add-ons, as desired.) Cover the top with the cheese.
11. Put the pizza directly to the oven rack. Bake for 10 minutes until the cheese is bubbling and melting from the center to the end. Let the pizza chill for 5 minutes before slicing.

Nutrition 242.8 Calories 15.1g Fats 15.7g Carbohydrates 14.1g Protein

22. Margherita Model

Preparation Time: 15 minutes

Cooking Time: 15 minutes

Serving: 10

Ingredients:

- 1-batch pizza shell
- 2-tbsp olive oil
- 1/2-cup crushed tomatoes
- 3-Roma tomatoes, sliced 1/4-inch thick
- 1/2-cup fresh basil leaves, thinly sliced
- 6-oz. block mozzarella, cut into 1/4-inch slices, blot-dry with a paper towel
- 1/2-tsp sea salt

Directions:

1. Preheat your oven to 450 °F.
2. Lightly brush the pizza shell with olive oil. Thoroughly spread the crushed tomatoes over the pizza shell, leaving a half-inch space around its edge as the crust.
3. Top the pizza with the Roma tomato slices, basil leaves, and mozzarella slices. Sprinkle salt over the pizza.
4. Transfer the pizza directly on the oven rack. Bake until the cheese melts from the center to the crust. Set aside before slicing.

Nutrition 251 Calories 8g Fats 34g Carbohydrates 9g Protein

23. **Portable Picnic**

Preparation Time: 5 minutes

Cooking Time: 0 minute

Serving: 1

Ingredients:

- 1-slice of whole-wheat bread, cut into bite-size pieces
- 10-pcs cherry tomatoes
- 1/4-oz. aged cheese, sliced
- 6-pcs oil-cured olives

Directions:

1. Pack each of the ingredients in a portable container to serve you while snacking on the go.

Nutrition 197 Calories 9g Fats 22g Carbohydrates 7g Protein

24. Stuffed-Frittata

Preparation Time: 10 minutes

Cooking Time: 15 minutes

Serving: 4

Ingredients:

- 8-pcs eggs
- 1/4-tsp red pepper, crushed
- 1/4-tsp salt
- 1-tbsp olive oil
- 1-pc small zucchini, sliced thinly lengthwise
- 1/2-cup red or yellow cherry tomatoes, halved
- 1/3 -cup walnuts, coarsely chopped
- 2-oz. bite-sized fresh mozzarella balls (bocconcini)

Directions:

1. Preheat your broiler. Meanwhile, whisk together the eggs, crushed red pepper, and salt in a medium-sized bowl. Set aside.
2. In a 10-inch broiler-proof skillet placed over medium-high heat, heat the olive oil. Spread the slices of zucchini in an even layer on the bottom of the skillet. Cook for 3 minutes, turning them once, halfway through.
3. Top the zucchini layer with cherry tomatoes. Fill the egg mixture over vegetables in skillet. Top with walnuts and mozzarella balls.

4. Switch to medium heat. Cook until the sides begin to set. By using a spatula, lift the frittata for the uncooked portions of the egg mixture to flow underneath.
5. Place the skillet on the broiler. Broil the frittata 4-inches from the heat for 5 minutes until the top is set. To serve, cut the frittata into wedges.

Nutritional   284 Calories 14g Fats 4g Carbohydrates 17g Protein

25. Greek Flatbread

Preparation Time: 5 minutes

Cooking Time: 10 minutes

Servings: 4

Ingredients:

- 2 whole wheat pitas
- 2 tablespoons olive oil, divided
- 2 garlic cloves, minced
- ¼ teaspoon salt
- ½ cup canned artichoke hearts, sliced
- ¼ cup Kalamata olives
- ¼ cup shredded Parmesan
- ¼ cup crumbled feta
- Chopped fresh parsley, for garnish (optional)

Directions:

1. Preheat the air fryer to 380°F. Brush each pita with 1 tablespoon olive oil, then sprinkle the minced garlic and salt over the top.
2. Distribute the artichoke hearts, olives, and cheeses evenly between the two pitas, and place both into the air fryer to bake for 10 minutes. Remove the pitas and cut them into 4 pieces each before serving. Sprinkle parsley over the top, if desired.

Nutrition 243 Calories 15g Fat 10g Carbohydrates 7g Protein

26. Vermicelli Rice

Preparation Time: 5 minutes

Cooking Time: 45 minutes

Servings: 6

Ingredients:

- 2 cups short-grain rice
- 3½ cups water, plus more for rinsing and soaking the rice
- ¼ cup olive oil
- 1 cup broken vermicelli pasta
- Salt

Directions:

1. Soak the rice under cold water until the water runs clean. Situate rice in a bowl, cover with water, and let soak for 10 minutes. Strain and putt aside. Cook the olive oil in a medium pot over medium heat.
2. Stir in the vermicelli and cook for 3 minutes.
3. Put the rice and cook for 1 minute, stirring, so the rice is well coated in the oil. Mix in the water and a pinch of salt and bring the liquid to a boil. Adjust heat and simmer for 20 minutes. Pull out from the heat and let rest for 10 minutes. Fluff with a fork and serve.

Nutrition 346 calories 9g total fat 60g carbohydrates 2g protein

27. Fava Beans with Basmati Rice

Preparation Time: 10 minutes

Cooking Time: 35 minutes

Servings: 4

Ingredients:

- ¼ cup olive oil
- 4 cups fresh fava beans, shelled
- 4½ cups water, plus more for drizzling
- 2 cups basmati rice
- 1/8 teaspoon salt
- 1/8 teaspoon freshly ground black pepper
- 2 tablespoons pine nuts, toasted
- ½ cup chopped fresh garlic chives, or fresh onion chives

Directions:

1. Fill the sauce pan with olive oil and cook over medium heat. Add the fava beans and drizzle them with a bit of water to avoid burning or sticking. Cook for 10 minutes.
2. Gently stir in the rice. Add the water, salt, and pepper. Set up the heat and boil the mixture. Adjust the heat and let it simmer for 15 minutes.

3. Pull out from the heat and let it rest for 10 minutes before serving. Spoon onto a serving platter and sprinkle with the toasted pine nuts and chives.

Nutrition 587 calories 17g total fat 97g carbohydrates 2g protein

28. Buttered Fava Beans

Preparation Time: 30 minutes

Cooking Time: 15 minutes

Servings: 4

Ingredients:

- ½ cup vegetable broth
- 4 pounds fava beans, shelled
- ¼ cup fresh tarragon, divided
- 1 teaspoon chopped fresh thyme
- ¼ teaspoon freshly ground black pepper
- 1/8 teaspoon salt
- 2 tablespoons butter
- 1 garlic clove, minced
- 2 tablespoons chopped fresh parsley

Directions:

1. Boil vegetable broth in a shallow pan over medium heat. Add the fava beans, 2 tablespoons of tarragon, the thyme, pepper, and salt. Cook until the broth is almost absorbed and the beans are tender.
2. Stir in the butter, garlic, and remaining 2 tablespoons of tarragon. Cook for 2 to 3 minutes. Sprinkle with the parsley and serve hot.

Nutrition 458 calories 9g fat 81g carbohydrates 37g protein

VEGETABLES AND SIDE DISHES

29. Moussaka

Preparation Time: 55 minutes

Cooking Time: 40 minutes

Serving: 6

Ingredients:

- 2 large eggplants
- 2 teaspoons salt, divided
- ¼ cup extra-virgin olive oil
- 2 large onions, sliced
- 10 cloves garlic, sliced
- 2 (15-ounce) cans diced tomatoes
- 1 (16-oz) can garbanzo beans
- 1 teaspoon dried oregano
- ½ teaspoon freshly ground black pepper

Direction:

1. Slice the eggplant horizontally into ¼-inch-thick round disks. Sprinkle the eggplant slices with 1 teaspoon of salt and place in a colander for 30 minutes.

2. Preheat the oven to 450°F. Pat the slices of eggplant dry with a paper towel and spray each side with an olive oil spray or lightly brush each side with olive oil.

3. Situate eggplant in a single layer on a baking sheet. Put in the oven and bake for 10 minutes. Then, using a spatula, flip the slices over and bake for another 10 minutes.

4. In a large skillet add the olive oil, onions, garlic, and remaining 1 teaspoon of salt. Cook for 4 minutes. Add the tomatoes, garbanzo beans, oregano, and black pepper. Simmer for 11 minutes, stirring occasionally.

5. Using a deep casserole dish, begin to layer, starting with eggplant, then the sauce. Repeat until all ingredients have been used. Bake in the oven for 20 minutes.

6. Remove from the oven and serve warm.

Nutrition: 262 Calories 8g Protein 11g Fat

30. Vegetable-Stuffed Grape Leaves

Preparation Time: 50 minutes

Cooking Time: 45 minutes

Serving: 8

Ingredients:

- 2 cups white rice
- 2 large tomatoes
- 1 large onion
- 1 green onion
- 1 cup fresh Italian parsley
- 3 cloves garlic, minced
- 2½ teaspoons salt
- ½ teaspoon black pepper
- 1 (16-ounce) jar grape leaves
- 1 cup lemon juice
- ½ cup extra-virgin olive oil
- 4 to 6 cups water

Direction:

1. Mix rice, tomatoes, onion, green onion, parsley, garlic, salt, and black pepper.

2. Drain and rinse the grape leaves.

3. Prepare a large pot by placing a layer of grape leaves on the bottom. Lay each leaf flat and trim off any stems.

4. Place 2 tablespoons of the rice mixture at the base of each leaf. Fold over the sides, then roll as tight as possible. Situate rolled grape leaves in the pot, lining up each rolled grape leaf. Continue to layer in the rolled grape leaves.

5. Gently pour the lemon juice and olive oil over the grape leaves, and add enough water to just cover the grape leaves by 1 inch.

6. Lay a heavy plate that is smaller than the opening of the pot upside down over the grape leaves. Cover the pot and cook the leaves over medium-low heat for 45 minutes. Let stand for 20 minutes before serving.

7. Serve warm or cold.

Nutrition: 532 Calories 12g Protein 21g Fat

31. Grilled Eggplant Rolls

Preparation Time: 30 minutes

Cooking Time: 10 minutes

Serving: 6

Ingredients:

- 2 large eggplants

- 1 teaspoon salt

- 4 ounces goat cheese

- 1 cup ricotta

- ¼ cup fresh basil, finely chopped

- ½ teaspoon black pepper

Direction

1. Cutoff the tops of the eggplants and cut the eggplants lengthwise into ¼-inch-thick slices. Sprinkle the slices with the salt and place the eggplant in a colander for 15 to 20 minutes.

2. In a large bowl, combine the goat cheese, ricotta, basil, and pepper.

3. Preheat a grill, grill pan, or lightly oiled skillet on medium heat. Dry eggplant slices using paper towel and lightly spray with olive oil spray. Place the eggplant on the grill, grill pan, or skillet and cook for 3 minutes on each side.

4. Pull out the eggplant from the heat and let cool for 5 minutes.

5. To roll, lay one eggplant slice flat, place a tablespoon of the cheese mixture at the base of the slice, and roll up. Serve immediately or chill until serving.

Nutrition: 255 Calories 15g Protein 15g Fat

32. Crispy Zucchini Fritters

Preparation Time: 15 minutes

Cooking Time: 20 minutes

Serving: 6

Ingredients:

- 2 large green zucchinis
- 2 tablespoons Italian parsley
- 3 cloves garlic, minced
- 1 teaspoon salt
- 1 cup flour
- 1 large egg, beaten
- ½ cup water
- 1 teaspoon baking powder
- 3 cups vegetable or avocado oil

Direction

1. Grate the zucchini into a large bowl.
2. Add the parsley, garlic, salt, flour, egg, water, and baking powder to the bowl and stir to combine.
3. In a large pot or fryer over medium heat, heat oil to 365°F.

4. Drop the fritter batter into the hot oil by spoonful. Turn the fritters over using a slotted spoon and fry until they are golden brown, about 2 to 3 minutes.

5. Take out the fritters from the oil and drain on a plate lined with paper towels.

6. Serve warm with Creamy Tzatziki dip.

Nutrition: 446 Calories 5g Protein 38g Fat

33. Cheesy Spinach Pies

Preparation Time: 20 minutes

Cooking Time: 40 minutes

Serving: 6 to 8

Ingredients:

- 2 tablespoons extra-virgin olive oil

- 1 large onion, chopped

- 2 cloves garlic, minced

- 3 (1-pound) bags of baby spinach, washed

- 1 cup feta cheese

- 1 large egg, beaten

- Puff pastry sheets

Direction:

1. Preheat the oven to 375°F.

2. Using big skillet over medium heat, cook the olive oil, onion, and garlic for 3 minutes.

3. Add the spinach to the skillet one bag at a time, letting it wilt in between each bag. Toss using tongs. Cook for 4 minutes. Once cooked, strain any excess liquid from the pan.

4. In a large bowl, combine the feta cheese, egg, and cooked spinach.

5. Lay the puff pastry flat on a counter. Cut the pastry into 3-inch squares.

6. Place a tablespoon of the spinach mixture in the center of a puff-pastry square. Fold over one corner of the square to the diagonal corner, forming a triangle. Crimp the edges of the pie by pressing down with the tines of a fork to seal them together. Repeat until all squares are filled.

7. Place the pies on a parchment-lined baking sheet and bake for 25 to 30 minutes or until golden brown. Serve warm or at room temperature.

Nutrition: 503 Calories 16g Protein 32g Fat

34. Cauliflower Steaks with Olive Citrus Sauce

Preparation Time: 15 minutes

Cooking Time: 30 minutes

Serving: 4

Ingredients:

- 2 large heads cauliflowers
- 1/3 cup extra-virgin olive oil
- ¼ teaspoon kosher salt
- 1/8 teaspoon black pepper
- Juice of 1 orange
- Zest of 1 orange
- ¼ cup black olives
- 1 tablespoon Dijon mustard
- 1 tablespoon red wine vinegar
- ½ teaspoon ground coriander

Direction

1. Preheat the oven to 400°F. Prep baking sheet with parchment paper or foil.

2. Cut off the stem of the cauliflower so it will sit upright. Slice it vertically into four thick slabs. Situate cauliflower on the prepared baking sheet. Drizzle with

the olive oil, salt, and black pepper. Bake for 31 minutes, turning over once.

3. In a medium bowl, combine the orange juice, orange zest, olives, mustard, vinegar, and coriander; mix well.

4. Serve at room temperature with the sauce.

Nutrition: 265 Calories 21g fat 5g Protein

35. Pistachio Mint Pesto Pasta

Preparation Time: 10 minutes

Cooking Time: 10 minutes

Serving: 4

Ingredients:

- 8 ounces whole-wheat pasta
- 1 cup fresh mint
- ½ cup fresh basil
- 1/3 cup unsalted pistachios, shelled
- 1 garlic clove, peeled
- ½ teaspoon kosher salt
- Juice of ½ lime
- 1/3 cup extra-virgin olive oil

Direction:

1. Cook the pasta following the package directions. Strain, reserving ½ cup of the pasta water, and set aside.

2. In a food processor, add the mint, basil, pistachios, garlic, salt, and lime juice. Process until the pistachios are coarsely ground. Add the olive oil in a slow, steady stream and process until incorporated.

3. In a large bowl, mix the pasta with the pistachio pesto; toss well to incorporate. If a thinner, more saucy

consistency is desired, add some of the reserved pasta water and toss well.

Nutrition: 420 Calories 3g fat 11g Protein

36. Burst Cherry Tomato Sauce with Angel Hair Pasta

Preparation Time: 10 minutes

Cooking Time: 20 minutes

Serving: 4

Ingredients:

- 8 ounces angel hair pasta
- 2 tablespoons extra-virgin olive oil
- 3 garlic cloves, minced
- 3 pints cherry tomatoes
- ½ teaspoon kosher salt
- ¼ teaspoon red pepper flakes
- ¾ cup fresh basil, chopped
- 1 tablespoon white balsamic vinegar (optional)
- ¼ cup grated Parmesan cheese (optional)

Direction:

1. Cook the pasta following the package directions. Drain and set aside.

2. Heat the olive oil in a skillet or large sauté pan over medium-high heat. Stir in garlic and sauté for 30 seconds. Mix in the tomatoes, salt, and red pepper

flakes and cook, stirring occasionally, until the tomatoes burst, about 15 minutes.

3. Pull away from the heat then mix in the pasta and basil. Toss together well. (For out-of-season tomatoes, add the vinegar, if desired, and mix well.)

4. Serve with the grated Parmesan cheese, if desired.

Nutrition: 305 Calories 8g fat 11g Protein

37. Baked Tofu with Sun-Dried Tomatoes and Artichokes

Preparation Time: 30 minutes

Cooking Time: 30 minutes

Serving: 4

Ingredients:

- 1 (16-ounce) package extra-firm tofu
- 2 tablespoons extra-virgin olive oil, divided
- 2 tablespoons lemon juice, divided
- 1 tablespoon low-sodium soy sauce
- 1 onion, diced
- ½ teaspoon kosher salt
- 2 garlic cloves, minced
- 1 (14-ounce) can artichoke hearts, drained
- 8 sun-dried tomato halves packed in oil
- ¼ teaspoon freshly ground black pepper
- 1 tablespoon white wine vinegar
- Zest of 1 lemon
- ¼ cup fresh parsley, chopped

Direction:

1. Preheat the oven to 400°F. Prep baking sheet with foil or parchment paper.

2. Mix tofu, 1 tablespoon of the olive oil, 1 tablespoon of the lemon juice, and the soy sauce. Allow to sit and marinate for 15 to 30 minutes. Arrange the tofu in a single layer on the prepared baking sheet and bake for 20 minutes, turning once, until light golden brown.

3. Cook remaining 1 tablespoon olive oil in a sauté pan over medium heat. Cook onion and salt for6 minutes. Stir garlic and sauté for 30 seconds. Add the artichoke hearts, sun-dried tomatoes, and black pepper and sauté for 5 minutes. Add the white wine vinegar and the remaining 1 tablespoon lemon juice and deglaze the pan, scraping up any brown bits. Pull away the pan from the heat and stir in the lemon zest and parsley. Gently mix in the baked tofu.

Nutrition: 230 Calories 14g fat 14g Protein

38. Baked Mediterranean Tempeh with Tomatoes and Garlic

Preparation Time: 25 minutes

Cooking Time: 35 minutes

Serving: 4

Ingredient:

For tempeh

- 12 ounces tempeh
- ¼ cup white wine
- 2 tablespoons extra-virgin olive oil
- 2 tablespoons lemon juice
- Zest of 1 lemon
- ¼ teaspoon kosher salt
- ¼ teaspoon freshly ground black pepper

For tomatoes and garlic sauce

- 1 tablespoon extra-virgin olive oil
- 1 onion, diced
- 3 garlic cloves, minced
- 1 (14.5-ounce) can no-salt-added crushed tomatoes
- 1 beefsteak tomato, diced
- 1 dried bay leaf

- 1 teaspoon white wine vinegar

- 1 teaspoon lemon juice

- 1 teaspoon dried oregano

- 1 teaspoon dried thyme

- ¾ teaspoon kosher salt

- ¼ cup basil, cut into ribbons

Direction:

For tempeh

1. Place the tempeh in a medium saucepan. Add enough water to cover it by 1 to 2 inches. Bring to a boil over medium-high heat, cover, and lower heat to a simmer. Cook for 10 to 15 minutes. Remove the tempeh, pat dry, cool, and cut into 1-inch cubes.

2. Incorporate white wine, olive oil, lemon juice, lemon zest, salt, and black pepper. Add the tempeh, cover the bowl, and put in the refrigerator for 4 hours, or up to overnight.

3. Preheat the oven to 375°F. Place the marinated tempeh and the marinade in a baking dish and cook for 15 minutes.

For tomatoes and garlic sauce

4. Cook olive oil in a large skillet over medium heat. Stir in onion and sauté until transparent, 3 to 5 minutes. Mix in garlic and sauté for 30 seconds. Add the crushed

tomatoes, beefsteak tomato, bay leaf, vinegar, lemon juice, oregano, thyme, and salt. Mix well. Simmer for 15 minutes.

5. Add the baked tempeh to the tomato mixture and gently mix together. Garnish with the basil.

Nutrition: 330 Calories 20g fat 18g Protein

SOUP AND STEW RECIPES

39. Squash and Turmeric Soup

Preparation Time: 10 minutes

Cooking Time: 30 minutes

Servings: 4

Ingredients:

- 4 cups low-sodium vegetable broth

- 2 medium zucchini squash

- 2 medium yellow crookneck squash

- 1 small onion

- 1/2 cup frozen green peas

- 2 tablespoons olive oil

- 1/2 cup plain nonfat Greek yogurt

- 2 teaspoon turmeric

Directions:

1. Warm the broth in a saucepan on medium heat. Toss in onion, squash, and zucchini. Let it simmer for approximately 25 minutes then add oil and green peas.

2. Cook for another 5 minutes then allow it to cool. Puree the soup using a handheld blender then add Greek

yogurt and turmeric. Refrigerate it overnight and serve fresh.

Nutrition: 100 calories 4g protein 10g fat

40. Leek, Potato, and Carrot Soup

Preparation Time: 15 minutes

Cooking Time: 25 minutes

Servings: 4

Ingredients:

- 1 - leek
- ¾ - cup diced and boiled potatoes
- ¾ - cup diced and boiled carrots
- 1 - garlic clove
- 1 - tablespoon oil
- Crushed pepper to taste
- 3 - cups low sodium chicken stock
- Chopped parsley for garnish
- 1 - bay leaf
- ¼ - teaspoon ground cumin

Directions:

1. Trim off and take away a portion of the coarse inexperienced portions of the leek, at that factor reduce daintily and flush altogether in virus water. Channel properly. Warmth the oil in an extensively based pot. Include the leek and garlic, and sear over low warmth for two-3 minutes, till sensitive.

2. Include the inventory, inlet leaf, cumin, and pepper. Heat the mixture, mix constantly. Include the bubbled potatoes and carrots and stew for 10-15minutes Modify the flavoring, eliminate the inlet leaf, and serve sprinkled generously with slashed parsley.

3. To make a pureed soup, manner the soup in a blender or nourishment processor till smooth Come again to the pan. Include ½ field milk. Bring to bubble and stew for 2-3minutes

Nutrition: 315 calories   8g fat   15g protein

41. Bell Pepper Soup

Preparation Time: 30 minutes

Cooking Time: 35 minutes

Servings: 4

Ingredients:

- 4 - cups low-sodium chicken broth
- 3 - red peppers
- 2 - medium onions
- 3 - tablespoon lemon juice
- 1 - tablespoon finely minced lemon zest
- A pinch cayenne peppers
- ¼ - teaspoon cinnamon
- ½ - cup finely minced fresh cilantro

Directions:

1. In a medium stockpot, consolidate each one of the fixings except for the cilantro and warmth to the point of boiling over excessive warm temperature.

2. Diminish the warmth and stew, ordinarily secured, for around 30 minutes, till thickened. Cool marginally. Utilizing a hand blender or nourishment processor, puree the soup. Include the cilantro and tenderly heat.

Nutrition: 265 calories   8g fat   5g protein

42. <u>Yucatan Soup</u>

Preparation Time: 10 minutes

Cooking Time: 20 minutes

Servings: 4

Ingredients:

- ½ cup onion, chopped
- 8 cloves garlic, chopped
- 2 Serrano chili peppers, chopped
- 1 medium tomato, chopped
- 1 ½ cups chicken breast, cooked, shredded
- 2 six-inch corn tortillas, sliced
- 1 tablespoon olive oil
- 4 cups chicken broth
- 1 bay leaf
- ¼ cup lime juice
- ¼ cup cilantro, chopped
- 1 teaspoon black pepper

Directions:

1. Spread the corn tortillas in a baking sheet and bake them for 3 minutes at 400ºF. Place a suitably-sized saucepan over medium heat and add oil to heat.

2. Toss in chili peppers, garlic, and onion, then sauté until soft. Stir in broth, tomatoes, bay leaf, and chicken.

3. Let this chicken soup cook for 10 minutes on a simmer. Stir in cilantro, lime juice, and black pepper. Garnish with baked corn tortillas. Serve.

Nutrition: 215 calories 21g protein 32g fat

MEAT RECIPES

43. Beef Corn Chili

Preparation Time: 8-10 minutes

Cooking Time: 30 minutes

Servings: 8

Ingredients:

- 2 small onions, chopped (finely)
- ¼ cup canned corn
- 1 tablespoon oil
- 10 ounces lean ground beef
- 2 small chili peppers, diced

Directions:

1. Turn on the instant pot. Click "SAUTE". Pour the oil then stir in the onions, chili pepper, and beef; cook until turn translucent and softened. Pour the 3 cups water in the Cooking pot; mix well.
2. Seal the lid. Select "MEAT/STEW". Adjust the timer to 20 minutes. Allow to cook until the timer turns to zero.
3. Click "CANCEL" then "NPR" for natural release pressure for about 8-10 minutes. Open then place the dish in serving plates. Serve.

Nutrition 94 Calories 5g Fat 2g Carbohydrates 7g Protein

44. Balsamic Beef Dish

Preparation Time: 5 minutes

Cooking Time: 55 minutes

Servings: 8

Ingredients:

- 3 pounds chuck roast
- 3 cloves garlic, thinly sliced
- 1 tablespoon oil
- 1 teaspoon flavored vinegar
- ½ teaspoon pepper
- ½ teaspoon rosemary
- 1 tablespoon butter
- ½ teaspoon thyme
- ¼ cup balsamic vinegar
- 1 cup beef broth

Directions:

1. Slice the slits in the roast and stuff in garlic slices all over. Combine flavored vinegar, rosemary, pepper, thyme and rub the mixture over the roast. Select the pot on sauté mode and mix in oil, allow the oil to heat up. Cook both side of the roast.
2. Take it out and set aside. Stir in butter, broth, balsamic vinegar and deglaze the pot. Return the roast and close the lid, then cook on HIGH pressure for 40 minutes.

3. Perform a quick release. Serve!

Nutrition 393 Calories 15g Fat 25g Carbohydrates 37g Protein

45. Soy Sauce Beef Roast

Preparation Time: 8 minutes

Cooking Time: 35 minutes

Servings: 2-3

Ingredients:

- ½ teaspoon beef bouillon
- 1 ½ teaspoon rosemary
- ½ teaspoon minced garlic
- 2 pounds roast beef
- 1/3 cup soy sauce

Directions:

1. Combine the soy sauce, bouillon, rosemary, and garlic together in a mixing bowl.
2. Turn on your instant pot. Place the roast, and pour enough water to cover the roast; gently stir to mix well. Seal it tight.
3. Click "MEAT/STEW" Cooking function; set pressure level to "HIGH" and set the Cooking time to 35 minutes. Let the pressure to build to cook the ingredients. Once done, click "CANCEL" setting then click "NPR" Cooking function to naturally release the pressure.

4. Gradually open the lid, and shred the meat. Mix in the shredded meat back in the potting mix and stir well. Transfer in serving containers. Serve warm.

Nutrition   423 Calories   14g Fat 12g Carbohydrates 21g Protein

46. Rosemary Beef Chuck Roast

Preparation Time: 5 minutes

Cooking Time: 45 minutes

Servings: 5-6

Ingredients:

- 3 pounds chuck beef roast
- 3 garlic cloves
- ¼ cup balsamic vinegar
- 1 sprig fresh rosemary
- 1 sprig fresh thyme
- 1 cup of water
- 1 tablespoon vegetable oil
- Salt and pepper to taste

Directions:

1. Chop slices in the beef roast and place the garlic cloves in them. Rub the roast with the herbs, black pepper, and salt. Preheat your instant pot using the sauté setting and pour the oil. When warmed, mix in the beef roast and stir-cook until browned on all sides. Add the remaining ingredients; stir gently.

2. Seal tight and cook on high for 40 minutes using manual setting. Allow the pressure release naturally, about 10 minutes. Uncover and put the beef roast the serving plates, slice and serve.

Nutrition 542 Calories 11.2g Fat 8.7g Carbohydrates 55.2g Protein

DESSERT RECIPES

47. Bananas Foster

Preparation Time: 5 minutes

Cooking Time: 6 minutes

Servings: 4

Ingredients

- 2/3 cup dark brown sugar
- 1/4 cup butter
- 3 1/2 tablespoons rum
- 1 1/2 teaspoons vanilla extract
- 1/2 teaspoon of ground cinnamon
- 3 bananas, peeled and cut lengthwise and broad
- 1/4 cup coarsely chopped nuts
- vanilla ice cream

Direction

1. Melt the butter in a deep-frying pan over medium heat. Stir in sugar, rum, vanilla, and cinnamon.

2. When the mixture starts to bubble, place the bananas and nuts in the pan. Bake until the bananas are hot, 1 to 2 minutes. Serve immediately with vanilla ice cream.

Nutrition: 534 calories 23.8g fat 4.6g protein

48. Cranberry Orange Cookies

Preparation Time: 20 minutes

Cooking Time: 16 minutes

Servings: 24

Ingredients

- 1 cup of soft butter
- 1 cup of white sugar
- 1/2 cup brown sugar
- 1 egg
- 1 teaspoon grated orange peel
- 2 tablespoons orange juice
- 2 1/2 cups flour
- 1/2 teaspoon baking powder
- 1/2 teaspoon salt
- 2 cups chopped cranberries
- 1/2 cup chopped walnuts (optional)

Icing:

- 1/2 teaspoon grated orange peel
- 3 tablespoons orange juice
- 1 ½ cup confectioner's sugar

Direction

1. Preheat the oven to 190 ° C.

2. Blend butter, white sugar, and brown sugar. Beat the egg until everything is well mixed. Mix 1 teaspoon of orange zest and 2 tablespoons of orange juice. Mix the

3. flour, baking powder, and salt; stir in the orange mixture.

4. Mix the cranberries and, if used, the nuts until well distributed. Place the dough with a spoon on ungreased baking trays.

5. Bake in the preheated oven for 12 to 14 minutes. Cool on racks.

6. In a small bowl, mix icing ingredients. Spread over cooled cookies.

Nutrition: 110 calories 4.8g fat 1.1 g protein

49. Key Lime Pie

Preparation time: 15 minutes

Cooking Time: 8 minutes

Servings: 8

Ingredients

- 1 (9-inch) prepared graham cracker crust
- 3 cups of sweetened condensed milk
- 1/2 cup sour cream
- 3/4 cup lime juice
- 1 tablespoon grated lime zest

Direction

1. Prepare oven to 175 ° C
2. Combine the condensed milk, sour cream, lime juice, and lime zest in a medium bowl. Mix well and transfer into the graham cracker crust.
3. Bake in the preheated oven for 5 to 8 minutes
4. Cool the cake well before serving. Decorate with lime slices and whipped cream if desired.

Nutrition: 553 calories 20.5g fat 10.9g protein

50. Rhubarb Strawberry Crunch

Preparation time: 15 minutes

Cooking Time: 45 minutes

Servings: 18

Ingredients

- 1 cup of white sugar
- 3 tablespoons all-purpose flour
- 3 cups of fresh strawberries, sliced
- 3 cups of rhubarb, cut into cubes
- 1 1/2 cup flour
- 1 cup packed brown sugar
- 1 cup butter
- 1 cup oatmeal

Direction

1. Preheat the oven to 190 ° C.

2. Incorporate white sugar, 3 tablespoons flour, strawberries and rhubarb in a large bowl. Place the mixture in a 9 x 13-inch baking dish.

3. Mix 1 1/2 cups of flour, brown sugar, butter, and oats until a crumbly texture is obtained. You may want to use a blender for this. Crumble the mixture of rhubarb and strawberry.

4. Bake for 45 minutes.

Nutrition: 253 calories 10.8g fat 2.3g protein

CONCLUSION

The Mediterranean diet is not just ordinary diet, but rather a way of eating that focuses on fresh, whole foods. It's not about restricting yourself or cutting out entire food groups, but rather eating fresh, seasonal produce, whole grains, nuts and seeds, and healthy fats – and cutting out processed foods and refined sugars. there are different research has been conducted on the Mediterranean Diet and it's been shown to reduce the risk of heart disease, type 2 diabetes, and Alzheimer's. People who follow the Mediterranean Diet tend to eat more fruits, vegetables, whole grains, nuts, seeds, legumes, olive oil, and herbs and spices. A Mediterranean-style diet is often associated with a healthy lifestyle and has been linked to a reduced risk of heart disease, cancer, and Alzheimer's disease. This diet emphasizes fruit, vegetables, whole grains, and healthy fats like olive oil, and it limits red meat, poultry, sweets, and junk food.

what you should do next is to set a small goal for yourself. For example, you can start with drinking a glass of extra virgin olive oil in the morning on an empty stomach. This way, you'll get used to the taste. You should keep track of your goal and how you are feeling each time you reach it.

If this is all too much for you right now, then just start with making one small change at a time until you get used to it.

As long as you do this and stick to the simple rules of a Mediterranean diet, you can attain all the benefits it offers.

another benefits of this diet is that it is perfectly sustainable in the long run, not to mention, it is mouth-watering and delicious.

Once you start implementing the various protocols of this diet, you will see a positive change in your overall health. Ensure that you are being patient with yourself and stick to your diet without making any excuses.

CPSIA information can be obtained
at www.ICGtesting.com
Printed in the USA
BVHW082029100521
606946BV00006B/1349